Tatiana Ryabtseva
Elena Sedelkina
Denis Makarevich

Contact Immunocorrection in in vitro experiments

Tatiana Ryabtseva
Elena Sedelkina
Denis Makarevich

Contact Immunocorrection in in vitro experiments

ScienciaScripts

Imprint

Cover image: www.ingimage.com

This book is a translation from the original published under ISBN 978-620-2-05520-8.

Publisher:
Sciencia Scripts
is a trademark of
Dodo Books Indian Ocean Ltd. and OmniScriptum S.R.L publishing group

120 High Road, East Finchley, London, N2 9ED, United Kingdom
Str. Armeneasca 28/1, office 1, Chisinau MD-2012, Republic of Moldova, Europe
Managing Directors: Ieva Konstantinova, Victoria Ursu
info@omniscriptum.com

Printed at: see last page
ISBN: 978-620-7-76254-5

TABLE OF CONTENTS:

CHAPTER 1

INTRODUCTION

The problem of resistance of pathogenic pathogens to antibacterial drugs was highlighted by the World Health Organisation back in 2001, when the fundamental document "Global Strategy to Contain Antimicrobial Resistance" was adopted and published (World Health Organisation, Geneva, 2001). The phenomenon of resistance of pathogens to therapeutic drugs, leads to a sharp decrease in the effectiveness of etiotropic therapy of recurrent infection. It is also established that polyresistant strains of pathogens to antibacterial agents simultaneously have increased resistance to the action of natural immunity factors [4]. Therefore, the means aimed at increasing the general resistance of the organism can currently be classified as the main ones used in the system of prevention and therapy of infectious diseases.

Today there are more than 200 names of immunomodulatory drugs, and the number of them continues to increase annually. [A.V. Karaulov, 2002.] However, the fact that taking drugs of immunotropic action has nuances of use, primarily related to the risk of developing hypo- or hyperimmune state, has been known for a long time and is much debated. In the best case, such drugs may not have any significant systemic effect due to the absence of direct contact of the drug with immunocompetent cells, and in the worst case, they may cause unpredictable reactions in the form of allergic, autoimmune reaction, immunosuppression, exacerbation of inflammatory process, manifestation of chronic infection, etc. [1,2]. [1,2]. In this regard, immunostimulants are reluctantly used for therapeutic purposes and favour the prophylactic administration of low doses, although such an approach not only does not reduce the likelihood of side effects, but also increases the probability of their occurrence. On the other hand, the growing number of research works aimed at studying the pharmacodynamics of the existing list of drugs for immunosuppression is justified, as they are widely used in oncology and organ and tissue transplantation.

In general, the growing popularity of immunopharmacology speaks not only about the increase in antibiotic resistance, but also about the urgent problem of treating the symptoms rather than the cause of the disease. Increasingly, researchers are finding that controlled stimulation of the immune system's internal reserves is sometimes much more effective, and almost always safer, than synthetic drugs with their myriad side effects. As a result, the need to improve the effectiveness of immune-stimulating therapy has pushed researchers around the world to search for safer, predictable and, at the same time, highly effective ways to adjust the activity of various parts of the immune system. Therefore, the development of methods of targeted cell specialisation, which implies artificial stimulation of natural functional reserves of the cell directed against a specific antigen, has become a natural development, and we will discuss it further.

This work is devoted to the search for new directions in immunopharmacology and the solution of existing problems. We will consider the possibility of using efferent therapy techniques as a tool for *contact* immunocorrection *ex vivo* and the creation of an experimental sample of medical equipment that will find its application in the therapy of various pathological conditions caused or accompanied by the presence of defects in cellular immune response.

CHAPTER 2
TARGETS AND MECHANISMS OF ACTION OF IMMUNOMODULATORS

Main groups of immunomodulators and their specificity

Currently, six main groups of immunomodulators are distinguished by origin: microbial, thymic, bone marrow, cytokines, nucleic acids and chemically pure [6].

Immunomodulators of microbial origin can be divided into three generations. The first preparation authorised for medical use as an immunostimulant was the BCG vaccine, which has a pronounced ability to enhance factors of both innate and acquired immunity. Microbial preparations of the first generation can also include such drugs as pyrogenal and prodigiosan, which are polysaccharides of bacterial origin. They are currently rarely used due to pyrogenicity and other side effects. Microbial preparations of the second generation include lysates (Bronchomunal, IRS-19, Imudon, relatively recently appeared on the Russian pharmaceutical market the preparation of Swiss production Broncho-Vaxom) and ribosomes (Ribomunil) of bacteria belonging mainly to the number of respiratory pathogens *Klebsiella pneumoniae, Streptococcus pneumoniae, Streptococcus pyogenes, Haemophilus influezae* and others. These drugs have a dual purpose: specific (vaccinating) and non-specific (immunostimulating). The third-generation microbial drugs include Lycopid, which consists of a natural disaccharide - glucosaminylmuramyl and a synthetic dipeptide - b-alanyl-B-isoglutamine attached to it. In the body the main target for immunomodulators of microbial origin are phagocytic cells. Under the influence of these drugs, the functional properties of phagocytes are enhanced (phagocytosis and intracellular killing of ingested bacteria increase), and the production of proinflammatory cytokines necessary for the initiation of humoral and cellular immunity increases [3,4,5].

Non-medicamentous methods of immunocorrection

Such methods include extracorporeal immunopharmacotherapy (EIFT) and additive immunotherapy, which uses controlled immunoregulation *in vitro. EIFT* is a cell-engineering method of immunocorrection, which allows the use of autologous immune response regulator cells *induced* in *vitro by* pharmacological drugs for the purpose of treatment and is used in the treatment of diseases of autoimmune genesis. Adoptive immunotherapy differs in that it is based on the transfer of lymphokine-activated cells or tumour-infiltrating cells into the patient's body [6].

The main advantages of EIFT are: the use of supratherapeutic doses of drugs that either do not enter the body or enter in trace amounts; contact of cells with pharmacological agent is strictly dosed in time; induced cells affect only physiologically targeted areas; it is possible to control the amount and degree of induction of cell function before administration [6].

One of the most controversial methods of immunocorrection is the use of monoclonal antibodies (mAbs), which bind to key receptors, improve antigen presentation, provide costimulation or counteract negative immunoregulation [7]. However, the use of drugs based on monoclonal antibodies is associated with the development of delayed-type hypersensitivity reaction, infectious complications (tuberculosis, viral hepatitis), lymphoproliferative diseases, leucopenia, thrombocytopenia and neutropenia [8]. In addition, one of the important disadvantages of monoclonal antibody treatment is the price.

Synthetic immunology is a new and most promising area of research that combines the latest knowledge and developments in molecular immunology and biotechnology. Research has led to the development of several elegant therapeutic strategies involving the synthesis of bifunctional molecules capable of intercepting antibodies against disease-causing cells and viral particles. These synthetic compounds, called ARMs (antibody-recruiting molecules), simultaneously bind to pathological target cells and have been shown to initiate antibody-mediated immune responses, including complement-dependent cytotoxicity, antibody-dependent cellular cytotoxicity, and antibody-dependent cellular phagocytosis of cell or viral particles [6].

Obviously, the idea of combining the advantages and efficiency of *in vitro* immunostimulation methods with the safety and selectivity of synthetic antibodies is very attractive. However, the high-tech and high cost of the described methods makes their use in the treatment of bacterial infections inexpedient. This gave the reason to start searching for a way to increase the efficiency of biological stimulators without resorting to expensive technologies.

The result of our research in this field is the *ex vivo* variant of cell stimulation. The method is based on the principle of immobilisation on a haemocompatible matrix of immunotropic objects, the search and development of which is carried out by the staff of the laboratory of haemo- and lymphosorption of the Belarusian State Medical University in cooperation with the specialists of the Institute of Bioorganic Chemistry of the IAS RB. The method is called *extracorporeal immunocorrection (ECI)* and consists in direct interaction of activator with target blood cells in the extracorporeal circuit. This method of *contact* activation relieves the method from the main disadvantage of EIFT - the need to extract target cells and incubate with the stimulant, which involves a number of technical difficulties and imposes restrictions on cell survival. Unlike traditional pharmacological agents, this method is not associated with the introduction of biologically active compounds into the body, so it does not require excretion of decay products and biotransformation, which allows the use of supertherapeutic doses for stimulation.

Various immunoactive compounds, both naturally occurring (proteins, bacterial cell wall components) and chemically synthesised (pharmacological agents, synthetic amino acid sequences, monoclonal antibodies), possessing specified physical and chemical properties with respect to target cells, can be used as ligand-activators in EI. The rapid development of biotechnology opens up opportunities for artificial reconstitution of necessary substances with specified properties, or changing the spatial structure of existing ones in order to improve or give them new properties. We are talking about synthetic peptide analogues that are able to mimic the activation signal in the cell by binding to the active centre of a receptor specific for a particular biological activator. Peptide ligands can be created depending on the specificity of the target object (receptor, protein, cell), activation or removal of which has pathogenetic significance for a particular pathological condition. It is also important that these technologies are not expensive, although they are more costly than ligands of biological origin (bacteria, fungi) and require highly qualified specialists in the field of molecular biology, immunology, biochemistry, biotechnology and medicine. Our specialists are currently conducting extensive research in this area and the preliminary data obtained give impressive results, which, we hope, in the future will open up new opportunities for the treatment of therapeutic, surgical, oncological diseases and some others.

Immune status of patients with chronic forms of purulent pathology.

In the emergence and development of chronic pyoderma, along with the peculiarities of the pathogen, its pathogenic, virulent and invasive properties, much attention is paid to the role of disturbances in the normal functioning and interaction of various parts of the immune system [9,10]. The bacterial factor in the body is counteracted by a multicomponent defence system, including innate (natural, non-specific) and adaptive (acquired, specific) immunity.

Non-specific factors of innate immunity constantly resist the impact of pathogenicity factors of opportunistic microorganisms, usually persisting on the skin and mucous membranes. However, when immune factors are weakened or when an excessive dose of even opportunistic microorganisms is ingested, the barriers of natural immunity may be breached and pyoderma may develop.

A complex of innate immunity factors can completely eliminate a pathogen without the development of a specific immune response. This complex includes cellular (macrophages, dendritic cells, neutrophils, NK cells, Tu/8, B cells, etc.) and humoral (natural antibodies, complement, acute phase proteins, some cytokines, lysozyme, etc.) factors.

Cells of the innate immunity system are widely represented in the skin and mucous membranes. A significant number of works have been devoted to the study of nonspecific defence factors in patients with pyoderma [11]. The main mechanism of antibacterial defence is phagocytosis. This is explained by the leading role of neutrophil dysfunction in the formation of recurrent or therapy-resistant infections, since neutrophils are the first line of defence against infectious agents. In long-term chronic recurrent pyoderma, there is a decrease in phagocytosis according to spontaneous and induced NST-test [12]. The data of electron microscopic study testify to the failure of neutrophils to eliminate infectious agents due to the absence or incompleteness of lysosomes [13]. The most studied neutrophil link in furunculosis and rye. There is a violation of absorptive and digestive function of neutrophils [14,15]. A decrease in the bactericidal activity of polymorphonuclear leukocytes in 47% of patients with recurrent furunculosis was found. When examining 150 patients with chronic furunculosis, 71% of them showed a decrease in the absorptive and bactericidal activity of phagocytes against Staphylococcus aureus [16].

Reduced bactericidality and impaired completion of phagocytosis are also reported by other authors. However, there are also reports about the absence of significant disorders in the neutrophil link. When studying the factors of non-specific resistance of the organism in rye, a high correlation between the activity of polymorphonuclear leukocytes and mononuclear cells and the severity of the course of the disease is also noted. The authors suggest predicting the course of rye at early stages using methods for determining the functional state of neutrophils [17].

In 67% of patients with recurrent furunculosis, an increase in the formation of reactive oxygen species by phagocytes under conditions of their metabolic reactivity (zymosan-induced luminol-dependent chemiluminescence) with no changes in spontaneous luminol-dependent chemiluminescence was observed. Thus, the absorptive and bactericidal activity of phagocytic cells is inhibited in pyoderma, which becomes one of the reasons for the severe course of the disease, often becoming chronic [18].

Increased susceptibility to bacterial infections is often associated with insufficient serum opsonising activity. Currently, the most important serum opsonins are considered to be the complement system and immunoglobulins. The participation of antibodies in the immune response manifests itself in three forms: neutralisation, opsonisation, and activation of the complement system. Antibodies contribute to the elimination of extracellular bacteria, ensuring the capture of the pathogen by phagocytic cells that destroy it in phagolysosomes. This process is accomplished through two pathways. In the first case, the pathogen coated with specific antibodies turns out to be much more accessible to phagocytic cells as a result of interaction of the Fc fragment of immunoglobulin with the Fc-receptor on the phagocyte surface.

The process of enhancing phagocytosis due to humoral factors in general and specific antibodies in particular is called "opsonisation". Only IgG antibodies have opsonising activity. Antibody-dependent cellular cytotoxicity is similarly mediated. It consists in the fact that foreign cells treated with IgG-antibodies die when co-cultured with leukocytes in the absence of complement. All cells carrying Fc receptors can participate in this reaction: neutrophils, monocytes/macrophages, B-lymphocytes, natural killer cells.

In another case, antibodies bound to the bacterial cell surface can activate complement system proteins that participate in a number of immunological reactions. First, by interacting with the pathogen, some proteins of the complement system act as opsonins, promoting, together with antibodies, a more efficient capture of the pathogen by phagocytes. Secondly, complement components act as chemotactic factors, attracting phagocytic cells to the focus of infection.

The third property of complement system proteins is associated with their ability to lysis some microorganisms by forming pores in their cell wall [16]. It has been shown that in the serum of patients with recurrent skin infection there is a deficiency of the C3 and C4 fractions of complement, which leads to impaired chemotaxis [17].

There are many mechanisms by which bacteria inhibit the functional activity of neutrophils and thus induce secondary infection. An example of mediated suppression is the incubation of human monocytes and lymphocytes with Staphylococcus aureus peptidoglycans, as a result of which these cells produce an inhibitor of neutrophil chemotaxis [19].

Low levels of opsonins accompany bacterial infections with severe or recurrent clinical presentation. Many bacteria have evolved defence mechanisms against opsonisation and subsequent phagocytosis by neutrophils. These defence mechanisms are mainly conjugated to the bacterial capsule. More than 50% of *S. aureus* strains isolated from patients are encapsulated. Components of the *S. aureus* cell wall *that* reduce the efficiency of phagocytosis are peptidoglycans and protein A, which binds IgG via the Fc fragment. The main component of the cell wall of another pyoderma pathogen, S. pyogenes, that prevents opsonisation is M-protein, which can be considered as the most important virulence factor. Staphylococci and streptococci produce exotoxins (leukocidins) that are lethal to phagocytes. For most capsular pathogenic bacteria, including Staphylococcus aureus and Pseudomonas bacillus, to which the capsule confers antiphagocytic properties, opsonisation with specific antibodies (mainly IgGl, IgG3) is a prerequisite for the efficiency of their phagocytosis via Fc-y receptors.

Both antibody concentration and affinity are important for effective antibacterial and antiviral defence. Antibody affinity is a qualitative indicator of the efficiency of microbial opsonisation. Changes in affinity may be the cause of decreased resistance to infectious agents. At insufficient concentration and low affinity antibodies are not able to have a significant bactericidal effect, which may be one of the reasons for recurrence of purulent-inflammatory process. When examining patients with chronic furunculosis, a pronounced decrease in the affinity of antibodies to the common antigenic determinant of all bacteria was noted in 14% [16].

Numerous studies point to disorders in the humoral immunity link [20,21]. The highest indices of humoral immunity, indicating a pronounced hyperproduction of all classes of immunoglobulins, were found in people with the first manifestations of furunculosis and rye and in persons with acute pyoderma. When studying the indicators of the humoral link of immunity in patients with pyoderma of more than 3 years' duration, a statistically significant decrease in the level of IgA and IgG and an increase in the level of IgM were found. In patients with furunculosis there is a decrease in the level of IgM on the background of increased concentration of IgG, in patients with chronic ulcerative pyoderma and vulgar ecthyma there is an increase in the level of IgM and IgG and a decrease in the content of IgA, while in patients with vulgar impetigo the indicators of humoral immunity were within normal limits. [22].

The authors find a correlation between immunological parameters and the stage, nature of course, duration, clinical form, etiological factor of the disease. In the phase of exacerbation of chronic furunculosis in patients there is a decrease in the absolute number of lymphocytes, lymphocytes with CD4 and CD8 markers (in 28, 59 and 21% of patients, respectively), a decrease in phagocytic index (in 14%) and an increase in induced luminol-dependent chemiluminescence (in 31%). In the remission stage, a decrease in total lymphocyte count (18%), CD3 (25%), CD4 (41%), and CD21 (19%) was found [23].

When examining individuals with various forms of pyoderma, the highest indices of humoral immunity, indicating a pronounced hyperproduction of all classes of immunoglobulins, were found in patients with the first manifestations of furunculosis and rye. Outside the exacerbation of chronic furunculosis, the indicators of cellular immunity were normal [15].

In patients suffering from chronic pyoderma for more than 3 years, changes in the indicators of cellular and humoral immunity, as well as in the phagocytosis system were observed. Statistically significant decrease in the level of IgA, IgG and increase in the content of IgM were in direct correlation with the content of B-lymphocytes against the background of a decrease in the number of T-lymphocytes, T-helpers and T-suppressors. Depression of the phagocytic system was revealed, manifested by a decrease in the number of leukocytes, neutrophils, monocytes, their functional and effector potential [24]. All this indicates the depletion of the organism's reserve capabilities in pyoderma. According to other authors, increased suppressor activity and suppression of activating function of T-cells, imbalance of some subpopulations of immunoregulatory cells are also noted in pyoderma [25].

Depending on the clinical form of pyoderma, types of changes in immune homeostasis are distinguished: marked activation of cellular immunity, characterised by an increase in the number of total T-cell population, an increase in the CD4 pool and an increase in the number of HLA DR-receptors on the membrane surface of T-cells in patients with staphyloderma. The activation of cellular link in pyoderma is reported in the studies of E.V. Novitskaya and S.A. Kovalenko [20]. The same authors point to a 4-fold increase in the number of NK-cells in patients with chronic pyoderma, which is considered a prognostic factor for chronicisation of the process. Other authors note an increase in the level of T-suppressors with an unchanged level of T-helpers against the background of a decrease in the absolute number of B-lymphocytes. N.H. Setdikova and T.V. Latysheva [14] point to the depression of the cellular immunity link by furunculosis in the form of a decrease in the absolute number of lymphocytes (in 33.3%), CD3 (in 31.7%), CD4 (in 57.1%), CD8 (in 23.8%), CD21 (in 26.9%). Also a decrease in the absolute and relative number of lymphocytes carrying CD3, CD4 markers and CD4/CD8 ratio against the background of an increase in the number of NK-cells was found by I.V. Gavrish et al. [24]. Other authors in the study of immune status in patients with chronic furunculosis did not reveal significant changes in the level of lymphocyte subpopulations [16], however, according to I.N. Gvozdeva, there was a decrease in CD4 content of less than 0.9 cells/l with normal other indicators of cellular immunity [26].

Depending on the severity of the course of pyoderma, for example, in furunculosis, the severity and nature of immunological disorders vary. In mild course in 70% of patients immunological indices are normal, in moderate and severe course there is a decrease in the absolute number of lymphocytes, lymphocytes with markers CD3, CD4, CD21 against the background of an increase in the level of CD8, which also indicates suppression of the cellular link of immunity. Some authors in the study of recurrent furunculosis in the exacerbation phase link the identified immunological disorders with the presence of concomitant pathology [22].

In ulcerative and ulcerative-vegetative forms of pyoderma there is a pronounced activation of the humoral link against the background of relative insufficiency of the cellular link in the form of a decrease in the number of CD3 and an increase in the level of CD21, IgA, IgG, IgM, CIC [27]. The same data were obtained when studying immunity in patients with pyoderma ulcerans and ecthyma vulgaris: almost all indicators of cellular immunity are reduced, there is dysglobulinaemia in the form of hyperproduction of IgM, IgG with decreased concentration of IgA. Other authors also report activation of the humoral link [28]. Many researchers emphasise the direct dependence of the depth of immunological disorders on the duration of the course of pyoderma. The deficiency of the T-system of immunity, as a rule, develops after 2-4 years and reaches a maximum by 10 years of the disease. In generalised streptoderma insufficiency of both cellular and humoral links was revealed.

Thus, when studying the immune status in patients with chronic frequently recurrent forms of pyoderma there is a marked activation of the cellular link of immunity, characterised by a significant increase in the level of leukocytes, the relative number of lymphocytes with markers CD4, CD8, NK-cells with normal indices of the humoral link. In patients with superficial forms with acute course there is a pronounced tendency of activation of humoral link in the form of hyperproduction of immunoglobulins against the background of increased level of CD21, CD22. In patients with deep forms of frequently recurrent pyoderma with a duration of more than 5 years there is a significant decrease in the relative number of lymphocytes, lymphocytes with markers CD3, CD4, CD8, CD22, C4 fraction of complement [29].

In the early 90's of the last century, a new direction in medicine, associated with the study of the mechanisms of regulation of intercellular interactions in the norm and in various pathologies, was intensively developed. By this time, the existence of a large group of polypeptide mediators involved in the formation and regulation of defence reactions of the organism - cytokines - was established. Cytokines are produced and secreted by cells of the immune system and fulfil the function of mediators providing intercellular cooperation, positive and negative immunoregulation [30]. Nowadays, more than 100 individual substances belonging to the cytokine family are already known. The significance of these proteins in the development of pathological processes and their role in the formation of the infectious process are discussed in numerous works, including those of a review nature. Most of the works are devoted to the study of the dynamics of proinflammatory cytokines such as ILip and tumour necrosis factor a (TNFa) content in blood in different infectious and infiltrative processes. Local production of TNFa in the focus of infection provides chemotaxis of granulocytes and monocytes into the focus, enhancing phagocytosis and phagocyte microbicidality. In response to infection, and as a result of the action of inflammatory agents on cells, increased production of PL occurs. Many proinflammatory effects of IL1, including participation in nonspecific anti-infection defence, are carried out in synergy with TNFa, IL6 [31].

Some of the strongest inducers of cytokine synthesis are components of bacterial cell walls: lipopolysaccharides, peptidoglycans, muramylpeptides. A typical inflammatory reaction arising in response to skin penetration by pathogens is formed with the participation of pro-inflammatory cytokines, which include PL, IL2, IL6, IL8, IL12, TNFa, u-interferon (IFNy). IL12 is an inducer of pro-inflammatory cytokines [32]. The development of inflammatory response is a factor involving adaptive immunity reactions, where the interferon family plays an important role. Among the functions of IFNY ONE OF THE most important is the activation of effector functions of macrophages: microbicidity and cytotoxicity, production of cytokines, superoxide and nitroxide radicals, prostaglandins. IFNy increases the expression of class 1 and 2 major histocompatibility complex antigens on the cell surface, thereby increasing the efficiency of antigen presentation and promoting its recognition by T-lymphocytes. IFNy stimulates maturation of medullary monocyte precursors, suppresses cytokine production by Th2 lymphocytes, and stimulates differentiation of TY lymphocytes. In staphyloderma, the IFNy content correlated with the duration of the disease, in streptoderma - with the severity of the disease, in streptostaphyloderma no correlation was found.

When determining the level of circulating idiotypic and anti-idiotypic antibodies to IFNy in the serum of patients, an inverse correlation between the content of anti-idiotypic antibodies to IFNy and the severity of the disease course was revealed [29]. Therefore, the use of recombinant IFNy in recurrent furunculosis is justified and gives a good clinical effect. The anti-inflammatory cytokine IL10 is an antagonist for IFNy. Bacterial cell wall components, including muramylpeptides, are strong activators of monocyte-macrophage system cells, which in turn, being activated, destroy pathogens by phagocytosis and formation of active oxygen radicals. Mononuclear phagocytes provide non-specific antibacterial defence of the organism not only due to their phagocytic function. Early pro-inflammatory and then anti-inflammatory cytokines secreted by them control the first line of defence against infections, providing recruitment and activation of macrophages, granulocytes, and NK cells. Peptidoglycan and its components can induce activation and stimulate the production by macrophages of cytokines - IL6, IL8, IL12, TNFa and IL1 - one of the main costimulators of T-cell activation, the main function of which is to participate in inflammatory reactions [33].

In recent years, it has been shown that IL12 is a key cytokine for enhancing cell-mediated immune response and initiating effective anti-infective defence [34]. The course and outcome of many infections depend on the ability of the pathogen, its components and products to induce IL12 synthesis. Selective inhibition of IL12 synthesis, even if the production of other proinflammatory cytokines (PL and TNFa) is preserved, allows pathogens to persist in the organism for a long time. The main effect of PL 2 is the induction of IFNy synthesis. IL 12 serves as an essential link between non-specific defence mechanisms and specific immune response. One of its most important effects is its ability to direct the differentiation of ThO lymphocytes towards ThY. In this effect it is a synergist of IFNy.

Pro-inflammatory cytokines are synthesised in the focus of inflammation mainly by macrophage cells. They are activated by cell wall components of pathogens and in response to tissue damage. Chemokines, which include at least 25 low-molecular-weight cytokines, in particular IL8 and R ANTES, enhance the migration of leukocytes into the focus of inflammation and, in cooperation with other cytokines, increase their functional activity [35].

Thus, at the local level cytokines are responsible for all stages of development of an adequate response to pathogen introduction. In case of failure of local defence reactions, an inflammatory reaction develops, cytokine synthesis increases, they enter the circulation and their effect is manifested at the systemic level. One of the vivid examples of severe hypercytokinaemia developed as a result of induction of IL1 and TNFa production by macrophages by bacterial endotoxin is bacterial-septic shock [36].

The study of such important immune effectors as cytokines in pyoderma patients has so far been fragmented, and in some cases contradictory data have been obtained. Recently, the role of cytokines in pyoderma has been actively debated. Few works devoted to the study of cytokines in pyoderma contain contradictory data and do not allow to determine the degree of cytokine involvement in this pathology. The development of pyoderma, like any infectious process, is accompanied by an increase in the concentration of the proinflammatory cytokine IL1. The following cytokines are the most studied in pyoderma: IFNy, IL1, TNFa, IL2, IL8. In a number of studies of cytokine profile in patients with pyoderma, depending on the stage of the disease, it was shown that in chronic furunculosis beyond exacerbation there are marked significant changes in the form of a decrease in induced production of IFNy, IL4, TNFa, IL8 and an increase in spontaneous production of TNFa, IL8, IFNy, which reflects the chronic nature of activation of the cytokine link of immunity. Disturbance of production of T-cell growth factor IL2, namely, an increase in spontaneous production, indicates persistence of the pathogen and the formation of secondary immunodeficiency. According to other authors, the average indicators of IL1 (3 and TNFa secretion in patients with pyoderma were significantly reduced [36]. However, the dependence of cytokine content in the vascular bed on the clinical form of pyoderma is noted: the lowest ILip and TNFa content is noted in patients with ulcerative-vegetative form of pyoderma, ecthyma vulgaris, conglobate acne, common sycosis and rye. In streptostaphyloderma and ostiofolliculitis (in superficial forms of pyoderma), ILip and TNFa levels are slightly higher with reduced IL2 secretion by mononuclear cells [37]. A correlation between serum IL8 level and NST-test parameters in pyoderma patients was found, which confirms the role of IL8 as the main chemoattractant and stimulator of biological activity for neutrophils. The diagnostic significance of cytokine level determination lies in establishing the connection of disorders with the course of the disease, in the possibility of predicting complications, as well as in the possible use of information about cytokines to assess the effectiveness of treatment. For example, it was found that antibiotic therapy is not accompanied by changes in the serum concentration of TNFa [38].

It is now recognised that the types of immune response are associated with one of the variants of lymphocyte activation with the predominant participation of helper T-lymphocyte clones TY or Th2, which differ in the set of cytokines produced and determine the direction of immune response development. Activation of Thy, secreting IL2 and IFNy, leads to stimulation mainly of the functions of T-lymphocytes and macrophages and the development of a cellular type of response, whereas the synthesis of IL4, IL5, IL10, IL13, IL25 by Th2 helper T cells stimulates mainly the humoral link [35].

In connection with the above, furunculosis is considered not as a local skin inflammation, but as a general systemic disease resulting from the development of predisposing immunological defects, often violating a number of important intercellular and biochemical interrelationships. Today, specialists all over the world are actively searching for new therapeutic methods, which not only more effectively fight acute diseases by affecting the pathological source, but are able to comprehensively stimulate or compensate for defects in natural adaptation processes in the human body.

CHAPTER 3

CONTACT IMMUNOCORRECTION

Nature of the active ligand for contact immunocorrection

It was decided to use fungal bioactive polysaccharides, which are, in our opinion, safer objects for medical use than bacterial ones, as an experimental sample of an extracorporeal immunostimulant. Indeed, some of the fungal cell wall biopolymers (mainly 0-glucan or heteropolysaccharide) have already found their place on the market as anticancer, immunostimulant or prophylactic drugs. [20]. Some fungi that are widely used today in traditional medicine as oral immunostimulants (baker's and brewer's yeast) can also be used for direct immunoregulation. An extracorporeal immunostimulant created using cell wall components of *Saccharomyces cerevisiae* (baker's yeast) will find its application in the treatment of secondary immunodeficiency states and chronic antibiotic-resistant forms of bacterial infection. Its potential application in oncology and rheumatology will be further investigated. However, the development requires thorough preclinical studies before this development can be transferred from fundamental to applied research.

Various compounds of natural origin (proteins, bacterial cell wall components) and chemically synthesised compounds (pharmacological agents, synthetic amino acid sequences, monoclonal antibodies) can be used as ligand-activators in EI. Despite the fact that activators of biological origin are strong immunostimulators of not only nonspecific but also humoral immune defence system, their use as ligands has a number of limitations. Due to their high immunogenicity, there is a risk of allergic reactions, hyperstimulation of cellular response, which can lead to quite serious consequences both for the immune system and the organism as a whole.

Therefore, it was decided to use fungal bioactive polysaccharides, which are, in our opinion, safer objects to use for medical purposes than bacterial ones, as an experimental sample of an extracorporeal immunostimulant. Indeed, some of the fungal cell wall biopolymers (mainly P-glucan or heteropolysaccharide) have already found their place on the market as anticancer, immunostimulant or prophylactic drugs [39]. Some fungi that are widely used today in traditional medicine as oral immunostimulants (baker's and brewer's yeast) can also be used for direct immunoregulation. The immunostimulator of extracorporeal type, created with the use of *mushroom* cell wall components, which is being actively developed by our laboratory staff, will find its application in the treatment of secondary immunodeficiency states and chronic antibiotic-resistant forms of bacterial infection. In the future, the possibility of its application in oncology and rheumatology will be investigated.

Changes in cytokine concentrations in blood of donors in response to exposure to active ligand *in an in vitro* experiment

Cytokines are small proteins (Mg 8-80 kDa) that act both on the cells that produce them and on surrounding cells. The formation and release of these highly active molecules are usually short-lived and tightly regulated. Cytokines play a central role in the positive and negative regulation of the immune response, as well as its integration with the physiological functions of other body systems - endocrine and haematopoietic. Recognition of microbial structures occurs at the very beginning of the organism's response to infection, before the development of a specific immune response.

The type of subsequent response depends mainly on the cytokines secreted. Different sets of cytokines secreted by effector cells activate their functions, but if inadequate effector function is activated, elimination of the pathogen does not occur and chronic immunopathology develops [30]. Our studies are aimed at the correction of such disorders. Thus, the study of cytokine-producing function should be a fundamental proof of the effectiveness of cell stimulation.

Table 1 shows the results of pro-inflammatory cytokine concentrations in supernatant after interaction of whole blood with yeast cell wall glycoprotein, zymosan and with viable baker's yeast cells.

As our studies have shown, the interaction of yeast glycoprotein and blood cells results in a statistically significant increase in the concentration of pro-inflammatory cytokines (TNF-a, IL-10, IL-6, IL-8).

Table 1 - Cytokine concentrations in the blood of practically healthy donors in response to activator action

Cytokine	P.R.	Glycoprotein	Yeast	Zymosan
TNF-a	13,59 (4,57;38,57)	274,69* (245,94;317,64)	345,14* (310,27;350,41)	5412,80* (2453,02;8372,58)
IL-10.	1,31 (0,00;13,62)	16,23* (2,13;62,36)	8,31 (5,59;17,61)	118,50* (7,02; 199,50)
IL-6	0,00	37,49*	8,49*	81,59*

	(0,00;3,56)	(24,81; 137,94)	(2,13;20,91)	(71,79;199,50)
IL-8	48,67 (35,77;187,80)	413,35* (399,35;498,00)	362,10* (275,30;386,90)	78,63 (67,49;89,14)

*- significant difference in pairwise comparison with control group (PE), $p<0.05$

For comparative evaluation of the intensity of the effect of different activators on cytokine production by neutrophils, the "I" coefficient was calculated. The intensity of the effect (I) was determined by the rate of cytokine synthesis per unit time and calculated by the formula: I= (Kl-K0)/t, where K1 - cytokine concentration after incubation with activator, KO - cytokine concentration after incubation with saline solution, t - incubation time.

The Friedman rank analysis of variance analysis of the data presented in **Table 2** showed that there was a significant difference between the rate of synthesis of different cytokines under the influence of different activators.

Table 2 - Rate of cytokine synthesis by donor blood cells in response to activator action (ng/min)

Cytokine	G lycoprotein.	Yeast**	Zimozan**	
TNF-a*.	2,55 (2,03;3,38)	3,06 (2,72;3,58)	57,86 (24,79;90,94)	p=0,0039 H=11,08
IL-10.	0,17 (0,00;0,68)	0,08 (0,04;0,10)	1,20 (0,07;1,52)	p=0,2181 H=3,04
IL-6*	0,41 (0,31; 1,27)	0,07 (0,03;0,20)	0,65 (0,28; 1,52)	p=0,0009 H=14,01
IL-8*	31,23 (18,66;50,82)	2,52 (0,65;4,24)	0,33 (0,00;0,94)	p=0,0243 H=7,43
Reliability of differences in the column	p=0,00738 к=1,00	p=0.04206 k=0.911	p=0.00635 k=0.850	Reliability of differences in the series

*- reliable difference between groups in the series (independent groups), we used the Kraske la-U o llysse rank analysis of variance

**-significant difference between groups in the column (dependent groups), Friedman's rank analysis of variance was used

Thus, when blood cells were activated with glycoprotein, the maximum synthesis rate was observed for IL-8 (31.23 (18.66;50.82) ng/min) *(Figure 1), and the* minimum for IL-10 (0.17 (0.00;0.68) ng/min). It should be noted that during the activation of blood cells by whole yeast cells the synthesis rate of all cytokines was insignificant, the highest value of the synthesis rate was observed for TNF-a, the lowest - for IL-6 and IL-10.

Under the action of Zymosan, blood cells synthesise TNF-a as efficiently as possible, while IL-8 synthesis is the least efficient. It can be concluded that whole cells of microorganisms activate cytokine synthesis insignificantly. While polysaccharides (Zymosan) or glycoproteins isolated from yeast cells providc active synthesis of cytokines by human blood cells. Moreover, activation of human blood cells by polysaccharides (Zymosan) leads to a significant accumulation of TNF-a (*Figure 2), while* activation by glycoproteins promotes the accumulation of IL-8 *(Figure 1).*

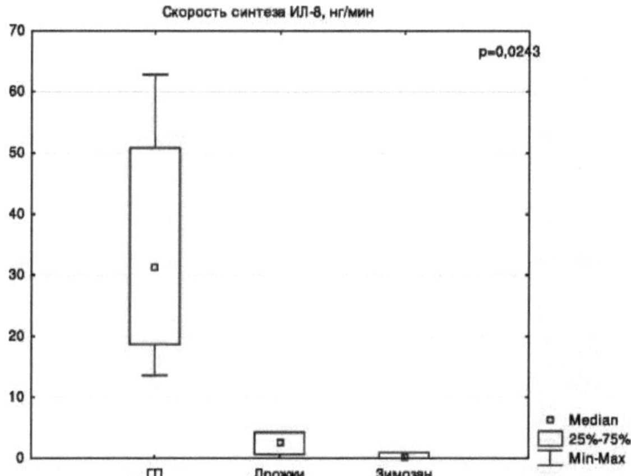

Figure 1 - Rate of IL-8 synthesis by immunocompetent blood cells under the influence of different activators.

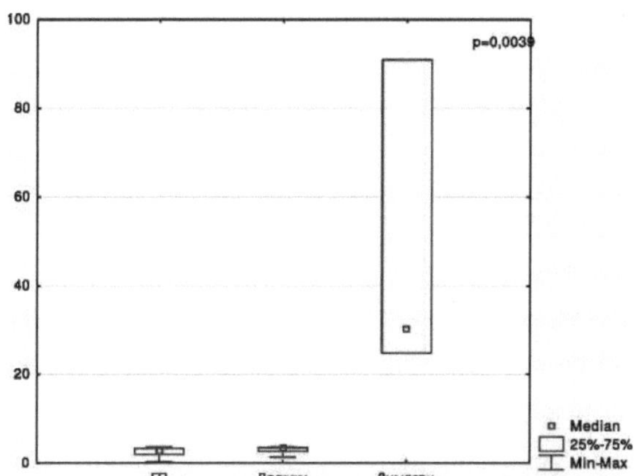

Figure 2 - Rate of TNF-alpha synthesis by immunocompetent blood cells under the influence of different activators

Given the severe systemic effects on the organism mediated by TNF-a [30], from our point of view, activation of blood cells by Saccharomyces cerevisiae glycoproteins is more preferable. IL-8 is a chemokine, promotes the expression of Toll-like receptors, which will lead to the activation of chemotaxis of neutrophils and monocytes to the focus of inflammation [35].

As for IL-4 concentration *(Figure 3), there* were no statistically significant changes in concentration. This fact indicates that the glycoprotein isolated from yeast cells activates to a greater extent blood granulocytes and does not affect lymphocytes.

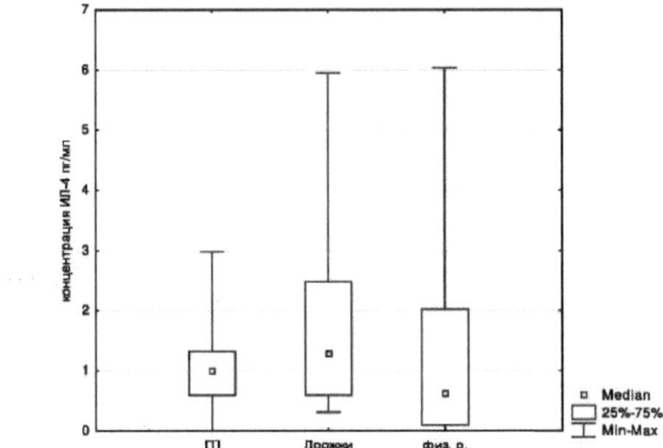

Figure 3 - Concentration of IL-4 in supernatant after contact of blood cells with activator

Thus, the glycoprotein isolated from yeast cell lysate has the ability to activate the production of proinflammatory cytokines by granulocytic blood cells, IL-8 synthesis is induced to a greater extent. After contact of blood cells with glycoprotein there is an increase in the concentration of TNF-alpha, IL-6 and IL-10.

Changes in leukocyte elastase and myeloperoxidase concentrations in donor blood in response to exposure to active ligand

Classical elastases are represented by three enzymes. Two of them belong to the class of serine proteinases: pancreatic and leukocytic elastase, and one belongs to the class of matrix metalloproteinases - macrophage elastase. During the development of inflammation and local pathological processes, leukocytic and macrophage elastases are the most active enzymes involved in intercellular matrix damage. Human leukocytic elastase is the main proteinase of azurophilic granules of polymorphonuclear leukocytes, which has a neutral pH optimum and has the most destructive effect on biological structures. Upon neutrophil activation, elastase is rapidly released into the extracellular space from the primary granules of leukocytes during their degranulation. In addition to its role in extracellular matrix degradation, elastase may function as a regulator of inflammation as it hydrolyses various anti-inflammatory cytokines such as IL-1, IL-2, IL-6 and TNF. Meanwhile, in the process of studying the biological effects of the activator, a significant increase in cytokine-producing function was detected and evidence of improved phagocytic activity was found, which could entail spontaneous degranulation of blood neutrophils and provoke the release of large concentrations of elastase under the action of the activator.

Thus, along with studying the concentration of cytokines in the supernatant, we studied the level of leukocyte elastase and myeloperoxidase. The results of the study are shown in Table 6. The median values of elastase concentration in blood with saline solution are around zero values, namely 0.09 (0.07;0.10) µg/ml. **(Table 3)** As expected, stimulation of phagocytic cells with live yeast cell suspension resulted in massive release of elastase into the extracellular space as a result of degranulation and phagocyte death (oxygen burst), which numerically represented 91.02 (33.99;152.42) µg/ml (*Figure 4).*

Table 3 - Concentrations of leukocyte elastase and myeloperoxidase (ng/ml) in supernatant after exposure to whole blood activator

Name	Glycoprotein	Yeast	Saline solution
Leukocyte elastase, µg/ml	0,15 (0,09;0,39)	91,02* (33,99;152,42)	0,09 (0,07;0,10)
Myeloperoxidase, ng/ml	23,35 (20,21 ;24,67)	24,85* (18,61;27,06)	17,16 (5,68;22,21)

* - statistically significant difference compared to saline solution

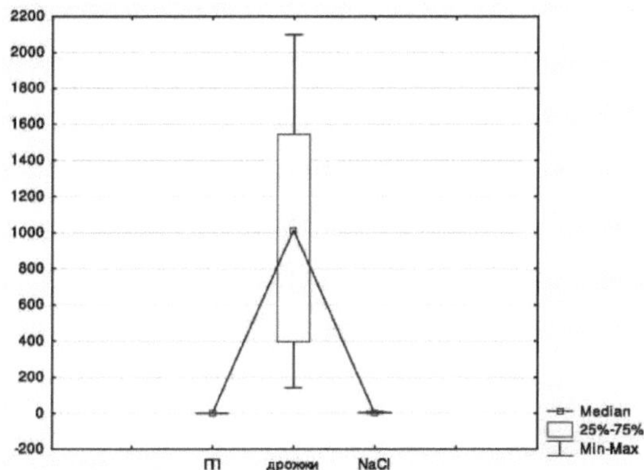

Figure 4 - Concentration of leukocyte elastase in supernatant after contact of blood cells with

activator (Friedman Method, p=0.00058)

No elastase release was recorded when cells were activated with the purified glycoprotein fraction: the median concentration in this case was 0.15 (0.09 ;0.39) μg/ml, which is comparable to the values in the control group **(Table 3).**

No significant change in myeloperoxidase concentration after blood contact with glycoprotein was recorded. Only in some cases we observed a significant increase in the concentration of myeloperoxidase in the supernatant after exposure of the investigated activators to blood cells. Similar results were obtained earlier when we studied the effect of glycoprotein on the change of elastase concentration. This conclusion speaks in favour of the safety of activator application in clinical practice, since damage to neighbouring cells and tissues, death of neutrophils and uncontrolled triggering of the inflammatory process are undesirable side effects of extracorporeal immunomodulation.

Changes in the expression of surface membrane markers on donor blood cells in response to exposure to active ligand

Table 4 - Changes in CD 177 expression on the surface of immunocompetent blood cells in response to glycoprotein action

Type of cells	P.R.	Glycoprotein
Neutrophils	87,80 (70,50;94,40)	99,20 (94,10; 100,00) *
Monocytes	1,85 (0,54;2,76)	4,80 (2,15;21,40)*
Lymphocytes	0,18 (0,09;0,46)	0,41 (0,22; 1,15)

* - statistically significant difference compared to saline solution

As shown by our studies presented in **Table 4,** after the interaction of yeast glycoprotein with blood cells of donors there is a significant increase in neutrophils and monocytes expressing marker CD177.

The CD 177 molecule is a human neutrophil-specific antigen. According to the scientific literature, the expression of this molecule on the surface of neutrophils increases under the influence of microorganism antigens and some cytokines [40].

There is also a hypothesis about the participation of CD177 in the development of microbicidal reactions of neutrophils. In addition, CD177 is a cell adhesion molecule that takes an active part in the migration of leukocytes to the focus of inflammation, mediating their interaction with endothelial cells. Thus, the isolated activator increases the percentage of neutrophils and monocytes capable of migration to the inflammatory centre through increased expression of CD 177

Cluster of differentiation CD 162 - glycoprotein ligand of P-selectin 1, PSGL-1 is a transmembrane protein on the surface of leukocytes, the main ligand of selectins. It plays an important role in the process of leukocyte retention and rolling on the vascular endothelial surface, the initial step in the binding, sequestration and transmigration of leukocytes during the inflammatory response.

The protein is found on neutrophils, monocytes and most lymphocytes [41]. Our studies showed that after the interaction of blood cells with yeast glycoprotein, the percentage of neutrophils, monocytes as well as lymphocytes expressing CD 162 decreased significantly **(Table 5). The** fact of decrease in CD 162+ neutrophils indicates cell activation. According to the literature, CD 162 expression decreases during the development of inflammation, as well as during activation by IL-6 and other proinflammatory factors [42].

Table *5* - Changes in CD 162 expression on the surface of immunocompetent blood cells in response to glycoprotein action

Type of cells	P.R.	Glycoprotein
Neutrophils	98,30 (93,90;99,90)	83,30 (59,90;92,30)*
Monocytes	98,70 (91,90;98,70)	93,90 (90,40;96,35)*
Lymphocytes	73,25 (67,20;75,60)	70,50 (53,20;72,85)*

* - statistically significant difference compared to saline solution

The results of studying the dynamics of Toll-like receptor (TLR) expression on the surface of immunocompetent cells are presented in **Table 6 and 7**. When *Saccharomyces cerevisiae* glycoprotein is exposed to blood cells, there is a significant increase in the percentage of both CD281+282+ cells and CD282+286+ cells (*Figure 5, 6, 7*). The increase in co-expression of TLR-1 (CD281) with TLR-2 (CD282), as well as TLR-2 (CD282) with TLR-6 (CD286) indicates the activation of neutrophils and monocytes, as well as their readiness to recognise antigens of gram-positive and gram-negative bacteria, as well as fungal antigens [43].

Table 6 - Changes in the expression of 281+282+ immunocompetent blood cells in response to glycoprotein action

Type of cells	P.R.	Glycoprotein

Neutrophils	0,67 (0,54;1,05)	1,43 (1,21 ;2,96)*
Monocytes	0,80 (0,51;4,06)	1,79 (1,14;11,10)*
Lymphocytes	0,16 (0,10;0,46)	0,12 (0,07;0,45)

Table 7 - Changes in the expression of 282+286+ immunocompetent blood cells in response to glycoprotein action

Type of cells	P.R.	Glycoprotein
Neutrophils	0,78 (0,51 ;3,06)	2,98 (1,33;8,66)*
Monocytes	1,02 (0,82;5,84)	1,84 (1,27;13,40)*
Lymphocytes	0,12 (0,11;0,45)	0,29 (0,17;0,38)

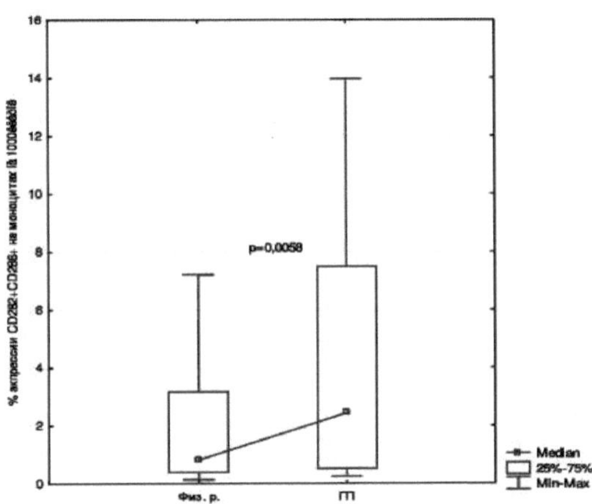

Figure 5 -Dynamics of 282+286+ blood monocytes in response to glycoprotein action

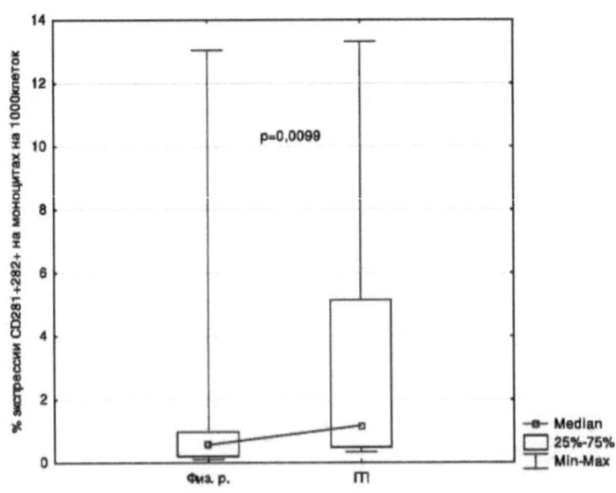

Figure 6 -Dynamics of 281+286+ blood monocytes in response to glycoprotein action

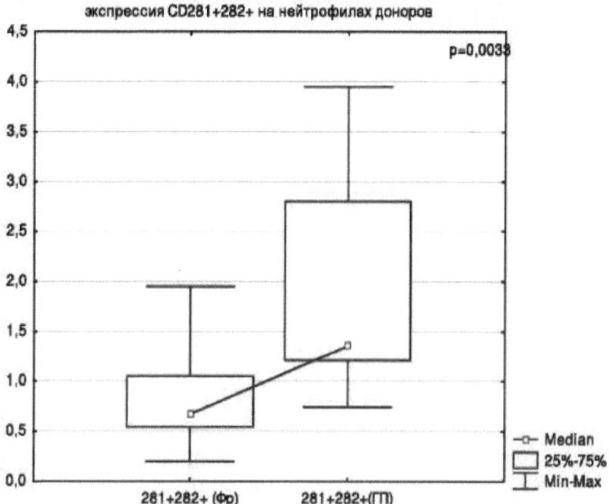

Figure 7 -Dynamics of 281 +282+ blood neutrophils in response to glycoprotein action

In the inactive state, toll-like receptors are monomeric in the membrane. Upon activation, they dimerise, leading to subsequent signal transduction inside the cell. Most receptors form homodimers, while for example THR-2 (CD282) forms heterodimers with THR-1 (CD281) or THR-6 (CD286) depending on the ligand. Our experiments showed a 2-fold increase in the expression of CD281, 282 and 286 on monocytes *(Figure 5, 6) and a* 3-fold increase on neutrophils *(Figure 7).* Activation of Toll-like receptors occurs upon binding of ligands, which for them are certain structures of bacteria, viruses and fungi. After ligand binding and receptor activation, the receptor binds in the cytoplasm to TIR domain-containing adaptor proteins, the set of which varies depending on the type of receptor and signalling pathway. For example, TLR- 3 binds to TICAM-1 (TRIF). TLR4 can interact with either MyD88 and TIRAP, inducing the synthesis of pro-inflammatory cytokines, or with TICAM-1 and TICAM-2, leading to the synthesis of interferons. Adaptor proteins bind to specific enzyme-kinases (IRAKI, IRAK4, TVK1 or IKKi) that significantly amplify signalling and lead ultimately to the induction of specific genes that determine the inflammatory response of the cell. In general, toll-like receptors are among the most potent cellular gene modulators [47,48,49].

CD69 transmembrane protein, a homodimer, consists of two highly glycosylated subunits with molecular masses of 28 kDa and 32 kDa and is a member of the C-type lectin family together with other members of this receptor family: NKG2, NKR-P1 CD94 and Ly49. CD69 expression is induced in vitro on most haematopoietic cells, including T- and B-lymphocytes, NK cells, macrophages, neutrophils and eosinophils, while it is constitutively expressed only on human monocytes, platelets and epidermal Langerhans cells [45].

Resting lymphocytes do not express CD69, but it is an early marker of activation that appears on the cell surface extremely rapidly. The density of its expression reaches its maximum in 30-60 min, and is detected 72 hours after cell stimulation. Note that the decrease in the density of expression almost ceases 8 hours after exposure.

Studies of CD69 expression on the surface of human and murine T cells upon stimulation with bacterial lipopolysaccharide (LPS) and TNF-a have been described in the literature. The analysis showed that early T cell activation is not solely dependent on ligand recognition via the T cell receptor (TCR), and that T cell activation independent of antigen recognition is probably a common phenomenon in infectious and autoimmune processes. It is likely that CD69 expression on T cells increases in response to subsequent TCR-ligand interaction [44].

In neutrophils, anti-CO69 monoclonal antibodies induce Ca influx^{2+} . Interestingly, this process does not require extensive binding of CD69 molecules. CD69 is also involved in lysozyme release and increases the expression of CD 11b on the membrane of PMA-activated neutrophils, suggesting a role for this molecule in the regulation of exocytosis [45].

De Maria et al. [66] report that CD69 acts as a potent signal transducing receptor also on human *monocytes*. CD69 binding induces Ca influx^{2+} and activation of cytosolic PLA2, synthesis of inflammatory mediators such as prostaglandin E2a, 6-keto-prostaglandin and leukotriene B4, which are released in equivalent amounts when monocytes are stimulated with LPS or cross-linking of CD69 with monoclonal antibodies, suggesting activation of cyclooxygenase and lipoxygenase. In addition, CD69 binding triggers NO synthesis and NO-dependent cytotoxicity of monocytes.

Thus, the study of CD69 expression on the leukocyte membrane provides information about the activation of cells under the action of activators of different nature at the early stages of stimulation. Our studies have shown that the percentage of neutrophils with CD69+ phenotype in the experiment after exposure to yeast glycoproteins reaches 81.90 (53.00;89.70)%, after incubation with physiological solution (control) this parameter was 64.20 (53.80;85.20)%.

However, the dynamics of CD69 expression on the surface of neutrophils was statistically unreliable. Multidirectional changes were observed in the course of the study. Most likely, CD69 synthesis and expression are mediated by different factors and depend largely on individual features of the organism. CD69 expression on monocytes after blood contact with glycoprotein decreased **(Table 8).**

Table 8 - Changes in CD 69 expression on the surface of immunocompetent blood cells in response to glycoprotein action

Type of cells	P.R.	Glycoprotein
Neutrophils	64,20 (53,80;85,20)	81,90 (53,00;89,70)
Monocytes	20,30 (2,87;31,10)	16,70 (3,61;32,50)
Lymphocytes	1,23 (0,40;8,68)	1,08 (0,57; 13,20)

As for lymphocytes, as noted earlier, CD69 is not expressed on resting lymphocytes. In the experiments performed, CD69 expression on lymphocytes was insignificant and did not change when the blood was exposed to the activator. This is a reason to believe that the selective effect of the isolated glycoprotein only on granulocytic cells.

Biological properties of immunomodule

The next step towards the creation of an extracorporeal immunomodulator was the study of an off-the-shelf haemoperfusion device containing an activator - an immunomodule. Immunomodule is a mass-exchange device filled with a *matrix* (polyacrylamide gel, polypropylene or polyethylene modified with acrylic acid) with a covalently *active ligand* sewn in. *The* study of biological effects of the immobilised ligand as well as the safety of its contact with whole blood are presented below.

Table 9 - Cellular composition of blood of donors after interaction with immunomodule

	Segment-eater	Lymphocytes	Monocytes	Eosinophils	Bacillus
Exodus.	57 (55;61)	37 (36;41)	3 (1;3)	3(1 ;5)	0 (0;1)
PAT	66 (58;69)	31 (28;39)	2 (1;4)	1 (0;3)	0 (0;2)
PAG + yeast lysate	62 (59;66)	36 (34;39)	1 (1;2)	1 (1;3)	0 (0;1)
PAG+GP yeast	59 (56;61)	38 (36;40)	0 (0;3)	2(1;4)	1 (0;1)

Table 9 shows the results of blood composition study of the field of interaction with immunomodule. As we can see, no significant changes were revealed.

Table 10 presents data of immunological indices of blood of donors after interaction with immunomodule. As can be seen, there is no change in phagocytic index. Some tendency to decrease phagocytic index after interaction of blood with PAG+yeast lysate was found. No changes in IL-6 concentration immediately after contact with the immunomodule were observed.

Table 10 - Changes in immunological parameters after interaction with immunomodule

	Phagocytic index, %	IL-6, nm/ml	IL-6, nm/ml After phagocytosis.	TNF-a, nm/ml	TNF-a, nm/ml After phagocytosis.
PAG	92 (92;96)	3,32 (2,95;3,70)	8,54 (7,15;9,94)	1,67 (1,13;5,15)	6,67 (2,13;8,15)
PAG+ yeast lysate	84 (79;87)	3,89 (3,07;4,72)	10,07 (8,92;11,23)*	2,33 (1,67;8,45)*	15,33 (5,67;28,45)*
PAG+GP yeast	95 (90;95)	3,39 (3,20;3,58)	11,90 (8,67;15,14)*	2,48 (0,34;3,89)*	27,48 (8,34;36,89)*

*- significant difference when comparing with PAG group, $p<0.05$

However, when adding microorganisms to blood (phagocytosis reaction) after its contact with the immunomodule, an increase in IL-6 concentration was observed compared to the sample after blood contact with an empty matrix. This indicates that when neutrophils contact with ligand (yeast glycoprotein, yeast lysate) their activation occurs and after addition of antigen (in this case live yeast cells) to blood a more pronounced immune response is observed. Similar results were obtained when studying changes in the concentration of TNF-a.

The activating ability of the developed immunomodule was confirmed by the change in the expression of activation markers on neutrophils and monocytes after donors' blood came into contact with the activating ligand sewn onto a polyacrylamide matrix **(Table 11,12,13).**

The percentage of neutrophils expressing CD281+282+ increased 4-fold after blood contact with the immunomodule. Thus, neutrophils become active and capable of antigen recognition after interacting with the ligand cross-linked to the matrix. Dimerisation of Toll-like 1 (CD281) and Toll-like 2 (CD282) promotes recognition of bacterial lipoproteins, peptidoglycans of Gram-positive microorganisms, and cell wall components of fungi.

Table 11 - Changes in CD 281+282+ expression on immunocompetent blood cells after

interaction with the immunomodule

Type of cells	PAT	PAG+GP yeast	PAG + yeast lysate
Neutrophils	0,44 (0,32; 1,64)	0,71 (0,58;4,69)	4,48 (1,63;6,71)*
Monocytes	94,6 (78,2;96,4)	97,0 (82,3;98,1)	98,9 (95,7;99,8)*
Lymphocytes	0,038 (0,022;0,065)	0,069 (0,041 ;0,098)	0,086 (0,082;0,093)
*- significant difference in comparison with PAT group, p<0.05			

Table 12 - Changes in CD 162+ expression on immunocompetent blood cells after interaction with the immunomodule

Type of cells	NAG	PAG+GP yeast	PAT + yeast lysate
Neutrophils	100,0 (96,3;100,0)	100,0 (94,1;100,0)	97,6 (96,7;98,5)*
Monocytes	90,9 (75,60;98,30)	83,4 (81,52;88,36)	84,7 (82,36;87,11)*
Lymphocytes	91,8 (90,2;96,4)	94,1 (91,1 ;95,3)	93,2 (92,6;97,3)
*- significant difference in comparison with PAT group, p<0.05			

Table 13 - Changes in CD 177+ expression on immunocompetent blood cells after interaction with the immunomodule

Type of cells	PAT	PAG+GP yeast	PAT + yeast lysate
Neutrophils	79,4 (75,3;81,6)	79,8 (76,0;88,2)	97,3 (95,8;99,3)*
Monocytes	47,3 (44,6;48,1)	53,7 (50,8;60,7)	58,3 (57,4;63,2)*
Lymphocytes	54,5 (53,1 ;59,8)	59,4 (55,8;64,1)	62,1 (60,7;65,9)*
*- significant difference in comparison with the ABO group, p<0.05			

After blood contact with the immunomodule we can expect an increase in chemotaxis of immunocompetent cells to the focus of inflammation, as our studies showed an increase in the expression of CD 177 on neutrophils, monocytes and lymphocytes of peripheral blood of donors, which according to literature data mediates chemotaxis of neutrophils under the action of some activators.

Effect of immunomodulator on cytokine synthesis by blood cells of patients with recurrent forms of chronic purulent pathology in response to stimulation by various activators in vitro

In order to be convinced of the ability of blood cells of patients with recurrent forms of chronic purulent pathology to respond to the stimulation of immunomodulators *ex vivo, the* following studies were carried out. Changes in plasma concentrations of cytokines and myeloperoxidase in response to stimulation of blood cells with yeast glycoprotein and zymosan were studied. Tables 14, 15, 16 present the results of comparative analysis of the effect of the investigated activators on blood cells of practically healthy donors and patients with chronic recurrent purulent infections.

The results of the study indicate a similar response of blood cells from patients and donors to exposure to activators such as glycoprotein and zymosan.

Table 14 - Effect of different activators on the ability to induce interleukin-6 synthesis by blood cells of patients with chronic suppurative pathology

Name	Glycoprotein	Zymosan	Saline solution
Donors	470,60* (304,64;611,46)	389,40* (333,20;603,80)	7,82 (0,00;1,88)
Patients	151,28* ** (47,06;352,16)	109,34* ** (51,23;265,48)	0,01 (0,00;0,01)

* - statistically significant difference compared to saline solution

** - statistically significant difference compared to the donor group

Table 15 - Effect of different activators on the ability to induce interleukin-8 synthesis by blood cells of patients with chronic suppurative pathology

Name	Glycoprotein	Zymosan	Saline solution
Donors	401,14* (397,58;425,58)	381,34* (321,58;405,34)	187,81 (48,67;303,01)
Patients	400,74* (388,01 ;427,03)	425,58* (334,21;489,32)	43,89 (8,72;130,38)

* - statistically significant difference compared to saline solution

** - statistically significant difference compared to the donor group

Table 16 - Effect of different activators on the ability to induce myeloperoxidase synthesis by blood cells of patients with chronic suppurative pathology

Name	Glycoprotein	Zymosan	Saline solution
Donors	23,35 (20,21 ;24,67)	24,85 (18,61;27,06)	17,16 (5,68;22,21)
Patients	25,15* (11,69;27,16)	27,85* (16,12;30,42)	8,40 (6,12;10,59)

* statistically significant difference compared to saline solution

** - statistically significant difference compared to the donor group

Thus, the glycoprotein isolated from the yeast cell wall can be recommended as a ligand for an immunomodule, which can be used in patients with chronic purulent infections to activate cellular immunity and suppress microorganisms in the focus of infection.

CHAPTER 4

CONCLUSION

The growing popularity of immunopharmacology speaks not only to the rise of antibiotic resistance, but also to the emerging problem of treating the symptoms rather than the cause of disease. Increasingly, researchers are finding that controlled stimulation of the immune system's internal reserves is sometimes much more effective, and almost always safer, than synthetic drugs with their myriad side effects. As a result, the need to improve the effectiveness of immune-stimulating therapy has pushed researchers around the world to search for safer, predictable and, at the same time, highly effective ways to adjust the activity of various parts of the immune system. Therefore, the development of methods of targeted cell specialisation, which implies artificial stimulation of its natural functional reserves directed against a specific antigen, has become a natural development.

The results of the safety and biological properties of the contact immunostimulant exhaustively prove that the ligand we created is an effective and safe contact immunostimulant of the nonspecific immune response. Contact immunostimulation will solve the problems of bioavailability and metabolisation and gives the possibility of using efferent therapy techniques as a tool for *ex vivo* immunocorrection. *In addition,* the method of ligand production and implementation of the treatment method is technologically simple and inexpensive compared to prototypes, which will make it in demand in the therapy of acquired immunodeficiency and antibiotic-resistant forms of chronic bacterial infections of different localisation.

In addition, the rapid development of biotechnology opens up opportunities to artificially recreate the necessary substances with specified properties, or to change the spatial structure of existing ones in order to improve or give them new properties. We are talking about synthetic peptide analogues of natural activators, which are able to mimic the activation signal in the cell by binding to the active centre of a receptor specific for a particular biological object. Peptide ligands can be created as an analogue of a receptor, protein or cell whose activation or deletion is pathogenetically relevant to a particular disease. These technologies are more costly than when using ligands of biological origin (bacteria, fungi) and require highly qualified specialists in molecular biology, immunology, biochemistry, biotechnology and medicine. However, our specialists are currently conducting extensive research in this area and the preliminary data obtained give impressive results, which, we hope, in the future will open new opportunities for the treatment of diseases of therapeutic, surgical, oncological profile and some others.

CHAPTER 5

REFERENCE LIST

1. Clinical immunology and allergology: Textbook / Edited by A.V. Karaulov. - Moscow: Medical Information Agency, 2002. - 651 c.

2. Immunodiagnostics and immunocorrection in clinical practice. - Edited by I.D.Stolyarov - Spb.: Sotis, 1999 - 176 p.

3. Dotsenko E.A., Rozhdzhdestvensky D.A., Yupatov G.I. Immunodeficiencies and some immunomodulating agents / Vestnik VSMU, 2014, Vol.13, No.3, pp.103-120

4. Novikov D.K. Immunocorrection, immunoprophylaxis, immunorehabilitation / 2006,198 pp.

5. Khaitov R.M., Pinegin B. V. Basic principles of immunomodulatory therapy // Allergy, asthma and clinical immunology. V. Basic principles of immunomodulatory therapy // Allergy, Asthma and Clinical Immunology. 2000, № 1, c. 9-16.

6. Sedelkina E.L., Ryabtseva T.V., Makarevich D.A., Bychko G.N.Kirkovsky V.V.. New prospects for the treatment of chronic bacterial infections using efferent methods of therapy / All-Russian scientific and practical conference with international participation, Ufa, 12-14 April 2016 //Fundamental and applied aspects of modern infectology, vol. 1. - C.228-234.

7. Juliet S. Gray, Peter W. M. Johnson and Martin J. Glennie. Therapeutic potential of immunostimulatory monoclonal antibodies // Clinical Science. 2006 Aug. No. 111(2): P. 93-106.

8. Aggarwal BB, Gupta SC and Ji HK. Historical perspectives on tumour necrosis factor and its superfamily: 25 years later, a golden journey // Blood. 2012, Jan 19. no. 119(3). P. 651-665.

9. Stulberg D.L., Penrod M.A., Blatny R.A. Common bacterial skin infections. Am Fam Physician, 2002, 66, l,c. 119-124.

10. Sharma S., Verma K.K.. Skin and soft tissue infection. Indian J Pediat, 2001, 68, 3, c. 46-50.

11. Lesnitsky A.I. Staphylococcal skin diseases (the state of various links of immunity and complex differentiated therapy): Avtoref. dis. dr. med. sciences. M 1986, 22s.

12. Shubin L.L., Lebedev V.A., Kokorev V.K., Kochetova V.I. On changes in nonspecific factors of organism defence and protein metabolism disorders in servicemen with

chronic pyococcal ulcers of the shin. Materials of the 15th scientific-practical conference of doctors. Nizhny Novgorod 1994, p. 129-130.

13. Rozum I.A. Derinat in treatment of patients with nasal furunculosis. Vesti otorinolar. 2002, No. 4, p. 12-15.

14. Setdikova N.H., Latysheva T.V. Complex mechanisms of development of chronic recurrent furunculosis and ways of their correction. Immunology, 2000, No.3, pp.48-50.

15. Kalinina N.M. Immunity disorders in recurrent furunculosis. Cytokines and inflammation, 2003, No.1, pp.41-44.

16. Karsonova M.I., Telnyuk Y.I., Setdikova N.H. Study of some features of immune status in chronic furunculosis. Immunopathol Immunol Allergol., 2002, No.3, pp.67-71.

17. Krasnova E.I., Mayanskaya N.N., Arkhipov S.A. Dynamics of spontaneous and stimulated NST-test of polymorphonuclear leukocytes in patients with rye. Homeostasis and infectious process: theses of reports of the international conference. Saratov, 1996,134 pp.

18. Dambaeva S.V., Mazurov D.V., Komogorova E.E., Setdikova N.H. Assessment of killer properties of phagocytising cells of peripheral blood in two groups of patients: with furunculosis and tuberculosis. Proceedings of the 4th National Congress of RAACI. M., 2001, No.2, p.59.

19. Totolyan A.A., Freidlin I.S. Cells of the immune system. St Petersburg 2000.

20. Novitskaya E.V., Kovalenko S.A. Possible prognostic markers of disease chronicity in pyoderma and furunculosis. Actual questions of dermatology and venereology. Moscow, 1997, p.118-119.

21. Baranova I.D., Molotilov V.F., Simonova A.V. Comparative immunological effectiveness of immunomodulators in the treatment of patients with furunculosis. Immunology, 1998, No. 6, pp. 18-19

22. Fazylov V.H., Kuklin V.T., Gilmullina F.S., Migranova G.M. Immunological aspects of the pathogenesis of swelling inflammation in combination with microbial eczema. Ros zhurn zhinn i ven bol., 2000, No. 5, pp. 13-14.

23. Chiller K., Selkin V.A., Murakawa G.J.. Skin microflora and bacterial infections of the skin. J Invest Dermatol Symp Proc., 2001, no. 6, p.170-174.

24. G avrish I.V., G avrish T.V., Zhuravleva T.V., Nechet V.A. Dysbacteriosis of

the skin, population and subpopulation composition of peripheral blood lymphocytes in patients with recurrent furunculosis. Med Immunol., 2000, No.2, pp.216-217.

25. Udzhuhu V.Y., Emuzova I.S. Dynamics of the main indicators of cellular and humoral immunity in patients with pyoderma in the process of monotherapy with viferon. Actual questions of dermatology and venereology. Moscow, 1997, p.148-149.

26. Gvozdeva I.N., Fedorov S.M., Rezaikina A.V. et al. Treatment of chronic pyoderma with helium-neon laser and immunomodulator ruzam. Vesti dermatol i venereol 1996;6:76.

27. Khoroshilova N.V., Kozyreva O.V., Simonova A.V., Setdikova N.H. Clinical and immunological characteristics of patients with chronic furunculosis. Congress devoted to modern problems of allergology, immunology and immunopharmacology, 3rd: Proceedings of RAACI. Moscow, 1997, p.451

28. Efremova V.N., Egorova N.B., Masyukova S.A., Gervazieva V.B. Effectiveness and reactogenicity of cell-free staphylococcal vaccine in immunotherapy of patients with chronic pyoderma. Journal of Microbiology, 1996, No.6, pp.39-41.

29. Volkova E.N., Butov Y.S., Morozov S.G. To the problem of immunopathogenesis of pustular skin diseases. Vesti dermatol i venereol. 2004, No.1, p.20-22.

30. Freidlin I.S. Paracrine and autocrine mechanisms of cytokine immunoregulation. Immunology, 2001, No.5, pp.4-7.

31. Simbirtsev A.S. Cytokines - a new system of regulation of defence reactions of the organism. Cytokines and Inflammation, 2002, Vol.1, No.1, pp.9-16.

32. Hodge-Dufour J. Inhibition of interferon-y induced interleukin-12 production: a potential mechanism for the anti-inflammatory activities of tumour necrosis factor. Immunology, 1998, T.95, no.23, p.13806-13811.

33. Asano T., McWaters A., An T. et al. Liposomal muramyl tripeptid upregulates IL-la, IL-10, TNF-a, IL-6 and IL-8 gene expression in human monocytes. J Pharmacol Exp Ther 1994;268:1032-1039Butakova, A.A. / A.A. Butakova [et al] // Immunology -1991. - №5. - C. 71-73.

34. Freidlin L.S. Interleukin-12 - a key cytokine of immunoregulation. Immunology, 1999, No.4, pp.5-10

35. Simbirtsev A.S. Interleukin-8 and other chemokines. Immunology, 1999, No.4,

pp.9-15.

36. Emuzova I.S. Immunomodulatory properties of interferon preparations in therapy of patients with pyoderma: Author's disc. candidate of medical sciences. M 2000

37. Korotkiy N.G., Emuzova I.S. Immunocorrection of leukinferon activity in patients with pyoderma. Vopr dermatovenerol i kosmetol. 1998, No.1, p.101.

38. Yaruta N.G., Kositskaya L.S. Cytokine profilc in patients with chronic pyoderma of different severity in the dynamics of treatment. Actual problems of fundamental research in biology and medicine. St. Petersburg: Nauka 2000, p.201.

39. Ioannis Giavasis. Bioactive fungal polysaccharides as potential functional ingredients in food and nutraceuticals. Review Article Current Opinion in Biotechnology, 2014, no. 26, p. 162-173

40. Ulrich J.H. Sachs, Cornelia L. Andrei-Selmer / The neutrophil-specific antigen CD177 is a counter-receptor for platelet endothelial cell adhesion molecule-1 (CD31) // The J. Of biological chemistry, V.282, No. 32, pp. 23603-23612

41. Zarbock A., Muller H., Kuwano Y., Ley K. PSGL-1-dependent myeloidleukocyte activation. J. Leukoc. Biol., 2009, no.86, pp.l 119-24

42. Hashizume M., Higuchi Y., Uchiyama Y. *I* IL-6 plays an essential role in neutrophilia under inflammation // Cytokine, 2011, N54, p.92-99

43. Iwasaki A., Medzhitov R. *I* Toll-like receptor control of the adaptive immune responses // Nature immunology, 2004, V.5, N10, p.987-995

44. R. Marziol, J. Mauel, S. Betz-Corradin. CD69 and regulation of the immune function. Immunopharmacology and Immunotoxicology, 21(3), 1999. P. 565- 582.

45. Risso, A., Smilovich, D., Capra, M.C., Baldissarro, L, Yan, G., Bargellesi, A., Cosulich, M.E., CD69 in resting and activated T-lymphocytes. Its association with a GTP binding protein and biochemical requirements for its expression, J. Immunol., 146: 4105, 1991

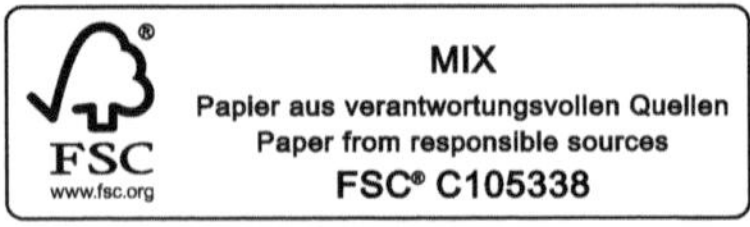

Printed by Books on Demand GmbH, Norderstedt / Germany